Healthy Gamer Lifestyle

Be your Game Avatar in Life

Lionel Thomas

Disclaimer

The information and advice presented in this book are meant to guide the reader in adopting healthier habits for a Healthier Gaming Lifestyle or other health achievements. Please, apply these well-known principles in a safe manner. The reader bears all responsibility for using or applying any techniques or ideas outlined in this book. Consult with your physician before starting any health or exercise programs.

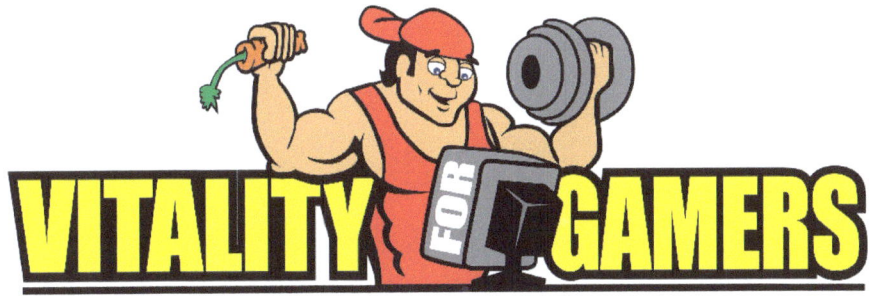

Brisbane, Australia.

www.VitalityForGamers.com

ISBN: 148021454X
ISBN-13: 978-1480214545

CONTENTS

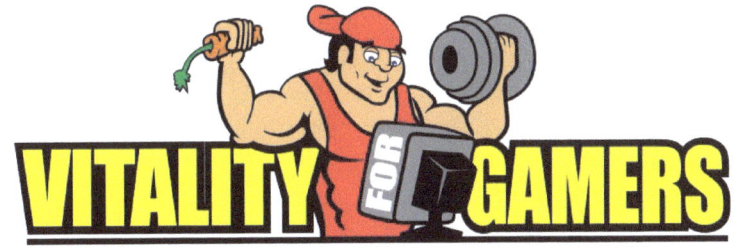

Birth of Vitality For Gamers

My name is Lionel Thomas; I am a Gameaholic and have been a computer Gamer for over 30 years. For the last 12 years I worked in the Computer Games industry, starting as a web programmer moving up to Games Producer, working on Xbox and PC titles.

It was Awesome! Working with games 40 hours a week, and then gaming at home for up to 60 hours a week, yes it is possible! Yet my body and health was degrading.

"If I could have been hooked up to a computer and play games 24/7, I would."

Over the years I ate anything, gained weight, had back problems, my health was poor and energy levels were like a rollercoaster (Moody as well). Most of this was oblivious to me, as I played out my life virtually with Role-Playing Games, First Person Shooters, Real-Time Strategies, MMORPG and much more… all that mattered was having my computer hardware working so I could play. Reality for me was to work so I could make money to buy games then play them.

Starting with only a few habits within 1 month I lost 5 kg (11 pounds); then over 8 months lost 20 kg (44 Pounds) improved my health, increased energy levels, became sick a lot less, regular and just felt great. **I explain how in this book!**

I play less virtually; yet play more in reality, as I am creating myself as my Game Avatar in Life. Part of this has been to create "Vitality For Gamers"; a cause to give computer Gamers increased reflexes, endurance and longevity for better gaming. In essence creating a 'Healthier Gamer Lifestyle' and changing the gamer stereotype.

The "Vitality Challenge" details the habits I created that made me realize that I could be my Gaming Avatar in Life. Since then, my Gaming and Non-gaming life have merged where anything is possible from here on in.

www.VitalityForGamers.com

"Be your Game Avatar in Life."

1. Gamer Risk

While computer Gamers spend hours fighting virtual enemies on digital battlefields, they face a very real threat to their health and safety; from muscle and joint issues to social balance, find out more about the potential threats to Gamer Avatars in life.

1.1 Fitness

University of Essex professor Dr. Dominic Mickle wright performed a series of tests on some competitive video Gamers to see just how they stacked up to what has been traditionally thought of as an athlete. The results of these tests proved shocking in both positive and negative ways in regards to the mental and physical health of the gamers.

> ➢ **Pros**
>
> The mental quickness and awareness of these gamers proved to be of a similar calibre to that of traditional athletes. In fact, some of the reaction time to changing visuals on the screen was even comparable to jet fighter pilots during war time. The Gamers also showed very similar characteristics to athletes in regards to how emotionally involved they become during times of heavy competition. Afterwards, they both feel accomplished and exhausted because of how taxing gaming and sports can both be, even though gaming requires basically no physical endurance. While these may seem like very positive traits, there is definitely a downside to spending so much time gaming.

> ➢ **Cons**
>
> The tests performed showed that the bodies of some of these Gamers were comparable to that of someone in their mid-sixties who had spent a lifetime smoking cigarettes. The

3

strength of their lungs was unusually low, which in theory is caused by the extreme lack of aerobic exercise. Other Gamers had bodies that seemed almost underdeveloped, like those of people much younger. The professor believes that such a sedentary lifestyle has hindered a lot of physical development traits, and he urges a balance between real life and the digital world.

Spending roughly ten hours per day in front of a screen of any kind can be very bad for a person's health, if they do not counteract that with some good physical activity and exposure to the sun. These tests show that there is a strong need for the human body to move around more and to become stronger under occasional physical duress. Doctors are saying that health problems, that used to never happen, are showing up in younger people, and this is allegedly due to the poor physical health of the video Gamer generation.

With so many people spending hours and hours per day looking at a screen, there is a need and duty for us to focus on some type of regular exercise regimen. It doesn't have to be running marathons or anything over the top, but it does need to be enough to keep us all healthy. Half an hour of aerobic exercise a few times per week is a great start. Technology is wonderful, but it doesn't do any good, if we aren't healthy enough to enjoy it.

1.2 Muscle and Joint Issues

Muscle and joint issues that are caused by the repetitive hand movements needed to play computer games. Increasing numbers of Gamers are being side-lined by real-life gaming-related repetitive strain injuries like muscle tears and nerve damage that can have some serious consequences for both work and play. Others have developed problems related to their musculoskeletal system like arthritis and sciatica as a result of their gaming habit.

What Is Repetitive Strain Injury & Carpal Tunnel Syndrome?
Repetitive strain injury (RSI) is a progressive condition that can affect the nerves, muscles and tendons of any part of the body that is subject to repeated movements for prolonged periods of time. Also known as isometric contraction myopathy, RSI usually affects the arms, elbows, shoulders, wrists and hands, leading to swelling, stiffness, pain and numbness.

Carpal tunnel syndrome is a painful, debilitating form of RSI that occurs when the nerve between the forearm and the palm becomes squeezed or pinched, leading to burning, itching and numbness throughout the fingers and hands. Initial symptoms can include a decrease in grip strength and dexterity. As this condition advances, many people feel like their fingers are swollen (despite the lack of visible swelling) and they lose their ability to feel temperature changes with their fingers.

What Causes RSI In Gamers?
Gamers are at high risk of RSI because most computer games involve repeated use of fine movements of the wrist, hand and thumb on a game controller, leading to overuse injuries and conditions like carpal tunnel syndrome. Because an injured muscle tends to shrink and contract, tiny tears develop in the muscle. Unless the muscle is rested and allowed to heal, continued use will lead to chronic pain and in some cases, permanent damage. Since most gamers play on a daily basis, any small tears and inflammation of the nerve passages that may occur tend to get progressively worse with time since rest is the key to healing these problems.

Other Muscle and Joint Issues Gamers Experience
Since most computer gamers play while seated, they are at an increased risk of developing problems related to poor posture such as herniated spinal disks, loss of muscle tone and arthritis. Gamers who have a poor diet and forego physical activity in favor of playing computer games are also at an increased risk of diabetes and obesity which can lead to problems with bone density, flexibility and overall good health.

Consequences of RSI and Gamer-Related Muscle & Joint Issues
Gamers who fail to seek treatment for RSI and gamer-related physical issues are at a high risk of developing lifelong problems that can leave them unable to play games, operate a computer mouse or even type on a keyboard.

1.3 Obesity

The issue of obesity among computer Gamers has been an emerging concern in today's society. Many people, young and old alike, find computer gaming a relaxing pastime mainly because it diverts their attention from typical daily stressors. However, sitting for long hours when playing computer games is actually a sedentary activity. Researchers believe that electronic games are associated with a higher risk of childhood obesity.

How Does Computer Gaming Lead to Obesity?

➤ **It promotes inactivity**
Unknown to many, sitting is a terrible habit that significantly contributes to having a fat physique. Statistics reveal that overweight people sit 2.5 hours more than people with average weight. Sitting down lowers a person's calorie burn rate to a measly 1 calorie per minute.

➤ **It encourages unhealthy eating**
Most Gamers tend to go for high-calorie snacks and junk foods which only add calories to their diet. Due to the absorbing

nature of most games, people find it hard to take a break and eat proper meals. Instead, they snack more on junk food and sodas.

➤ **It replaces outdoor games**
Children, and even adults, may prefer playing computer games rather than experiencing healthy physical outdoor activities. They choose to play games for many hours leaving no time for sports.

According to researchers at Bristol University and Loughborough University, a sedentary lifestyle that's linked to spending too much time playing computer games may increase the risk of obesity considering that electronic game playing involves little physical activity.

Studies also show that obese gamers may experience the following effects:

➤ **Higher risk for serious health conditions**
Obese people are prone to serious health problems such as high blood pressure, cardiac diseases, high cholesterol, and type 2 diabetes. Although these diseases used to be considered exclusive to adults, youngsters today, especially those who don't have a healthy lifestyle, are already vulnerable to such serious medical conditions. Other medical effects of obesity include bone and joint problems, eating disorders, disordered sleep patterns, liver disease, breathing difficulties, and depression.

➤ **Causes bad posture**
Experts say that obesity leads to bad posture as it forces the spine out of alignment in an attempt to distribute excess weight evenly and to keep the body upright. This increases stress on the vertebrae, muscles, and ligaments. Bad posture worsens as the curve in the lower back increases, and this is prevalent in obese Gamers.

➤ **Causes back pain**
Obese gamers suffer more easily from back pain while staying in a sedentary sitting position during game play. This hampers their gaming experience and causes more difficulty in playing games for prolonged periods.

➤ **Leads to slower body performance**
Overweight people are more likely to suffer from breathing problems during intense activities. For Gamers, having extra weight means slower bodily movements and response time.

➤ **Psychosocial Effects**
In a culture where the general idea of physical attractiveness is a slim physique, overweight people may suffer from low self-esteem and a poor social life. This pushes them to seclude themselves from others and indulge more in electronic gaming rather than socializing.

Obese kids and teens have a higher possibility of developing chronic health conditions in their later years; thus, it's important to prevent obesity early on. For avid computer gaming enthusiasts, it's best to exert more control over their gaming habit. Setting time limitations, as well as engaging in healthy activities, such as exercising are highly recommended.

1.4 Eye Strain

Today's computer games are filled with rapid movements and mind-blowing visual effects, with newer games even offering 3-D features. To really enjoy playing, Gamers need to have healthy eyes; however, many Gamers suffer from vision problems related to gaming known as "Gamer Eye Strain", also known as "Computer Vision Syndrome". Left untreated, this condition can leave Gamers unable to react to visual game cues, and in extreme cases, some Gamers are unable to even look at a computer screen unassisted.

What Is Gamer Eye Strain?

Gamer eye strain is a condition that occurs when a Gamer develops problems with their vision as a result of prolonged gaming. Playing video games is demanding on the eyes, requiring the muscles in the eyes to constantly work to refocus and adjust to rapid changes in lighting and movement for extended periods of time; in addition to the focal point being nearly the same distance the whole time. Gamer Eye Strain is considered to be a repetitive strain injury, similar to other conditions like carpal tunnel syndrome that are caused by overuse of a particular muscle or group of muscles.

Symptoms of Gamer Eye Strain

This condition can cause a number of uncomfortable symptoms including:

- ➤ The inability to focus on fine movements and small objects.
- ➤ Pain throughout the neck and upper back.
- ➤ Headaches and nausea.
- ➤ Red, irritated eyes.
- ➤ Double vision and impaired night vision.
- ➤ Reduced reaction times while driving, gaming and playing sports.
- ➤ Pain throughout the eyes and head when viewing a screen such as a computer monitor, TV or smartphone.

Who Is At Risk?

Anyone who spends time playing computer games is at risk of developing gamer eye strain. This risk increases relative to amount of time spent gaming along with time spent in front of a computer screen working or surfing the web. Adding other types of 'screen time' such as watching TV, going to the movies or using a smartphone also increases the risk of developing gamer eye strain.

Gamers who have pre-existing vision problems such as an astigmatism tend to develop computer vision syndrome faster than Gamers who have 20/20 vision, and those who are over the age of 40 also face an increased risk of developing this condition. As people age, their ability to focus on objects that are either too close or too far away diminishes, adding to the amount of work the muscles of the eye need to do to focus on a computer screen.

Consequences & Complications Of Gamer Eye Strain

While Gamer Eye Strain has not been linked to any long-term health consequences it can have a significant, negative impact on day-to-day life. Gamers who work on computers all day risk losing their ability to work if the symptoms of computer vision syndrome go untreated, while daily activities such as operating a motorized vehicle can become extremely dangerous for those with gaming-related blurry vision and eye problems. Students who have gamer eye strain often have difficulties attending school and completing homework, while people of all ages can become lethargic and sedentary when vision problems restrict their ability to enjoy physical and social activities.

1.5 Gameaholism

There have been numerous studies done on the effects of video games on children and teenagers, particularly when it comes to violence and how that may affect behavior. It has been shown that video games can affect the growing brain in both beneficial and harmful ways, correlating to the type of games played as well as the frequency and duration of the gameplay. Finally, researchers are beginning to research the effects of prolonged video gaming on adults and what they're discovering is not good news.

Although the American Medical Association has yet to officially recognize video game addiction "**Gameaholism**" as a psychiatric condition, many experts agree that there is a strong potential for pathological addiction; to become a "**Gameholic**". The effects on the brain are the same as that of gambling addiction and very similar to drug and alcohol addiction. Risks of several health issues increase with excessive time spent gaming, whether on a console or on the computer.

One of the first major studies to be done on adult gamers was led by James Weaver with the Center for Disease Control and National Center for Health Marketing. The study subjects were 562 adults between the ages of 19 and 90, all living in Washington. Of those subjects, 45.1% said they play video games on a regular basis.

Social Balance

The study showed that female gamers had more incidents of depression and lower health status than non-gaming females, while men showed increased likelihood of increased body mass index. Both genders indicated that excessive gaming increased the players dependence on the internet for socializing. The study also showed a significant decrease in sociability levels the more hours the subject spent gaming.

It's not surprising to see that sociability is affected by excessive gaming. Many previous studies, while done on young people, have indicated that overdoing video games leads to lower attention spans, higher levels of aggression, less social interaction and depression. All of these symptoms could have a strong impact on gamer social balance.

Those with video game addiction "Gameaholics", often cut themselves off from social interactions or find that they cannot maintain their attention on others. This imbalance isolates the game addict and can lead to loneliness and depression.

1.6 Kid Gamers

Despite what horror movies have tried to teach us, it does not take experimental viruses, cosmic radiation, or black magic to make zombies. Instead, all you have to do is put a video game within reach of a child. In no time at all you'll have a glazed, open-mouthed unresponsive zombie. Since video games were invented, children have started spending more and more time playing video games and less and less time doing almost anything else. This could be causing health problems, of both physical and mental varieties. When deciding whether or not to allow your kids to play video games, or how much to allow them to play, you need to look closely at the pros and cons.

Many of these games have a lot of gore in them, as well as suggestive themes. Some studies seem to suggest that prolonged exposure to violent video games makes kids more accepting of violence, although nothing conclusive has been proven. So the question remains open. Will violent video games make your kids violent?

> ➢ **Pros**

Video games have many positive benefits for children. They give the brain a workout, and teach valuable problem solving skills. While your kid may look like a zombie while gaming, in fact he or she is actually learning. Some video games are so complex and challenging that they require truly high level thinking in order to master them, and learning this kind of thinking has benefits that your kids will be able to apply later in life in many different ways. Video games also develop hand-eye coordination, motor skills, and spatial skills.

Video games also teach children about computer technology and the Internet. Computers are a major part of life in the modern world, and familiarity with them at a young age will be of benefit to their future careers. They can also help your family bond. Many video games are meant to be played by multiple people at once. Some video games are even built around furthering a child's education.

➤ Cons

Excessive play of video games can make your child socially isolated. Video games can be addictive, and the need to beat a game can cause children to neglect social activities and ignore their friends and family. It can also cause children to neglect their homework, reading, and sports.

Some video games can teach inappropriate values as well. Women are often portrayed as weak or useless. Players are often encouraged to do violent, inappropriate, and even outright evil things.

Video game addiction can cause your child's grades to fall. They can also cause their health to suffer. The more they stay inside playing video games, the less they are outside getting exercise. This can lead to weakness, obesity, carpal tunnel syndrome, and more.

2. Healthy Gamer

2.1 Habit Creation

When people talk about habits, they almost always refer to bad habits that they feel they must change but very little discussion is heard about good habits. A habit is nothing more than learned behaviors that have become so engrained in the thought patterns that the behaviors become automatic and you no longer consciously think about it. These patterns can be either beneficial or detrimental.

Most of the time, habit creation is done unintentionally and you don't even realize you're doing it until the habit is established but this doesn't have to be the case. Once you are aware of any detrimental habit, you can purposely re-create those thought patterns to eliminate the undesirable habit. You can also purposely create a desirable habit by following the steps below.

Steps to Healthy Habit Creation

When it comes to creating healthy habits, there are really only two main steps. You need to formulate a plan and make a deep commitment to following through on that plan.

1. **Plan**

   What healthy habits do you want to create? Make a list of all that you can think of and then prioritize your list by which habits will make the biggest change for you.

   Which of those habits would provide the most benefit to you right now? That is the habit you want to focus on first. Choose only one habit at a time to focus on.

Be specific with what you want. If you wish to get in the habit of working out, don't state your goal as "work out every day." Instead, state something like, "work out 20 minutes each morning before starting my work."

Write this specific goal out. **The act of writing stimulates sectors in the brain and imprints it on your mind better** than just saying it would. It combines the thoughts, actions and visual center of the brain. Your brain will unconsciously work to help you achieve this goal once it's imprinted in your psyche.

2. Commitment

You must be totally committed to creating this habit until it's fully formed. Habits are not formed in only a few days. Commit to at least 30 days, as studies have shown that **it takes at least 21 times of doing something in a row to form a lasting habit.**

Remember, though, research results are averages and what the majority achieves. Everyone is different and you could form a habit in less time or take twice as long. Just remember that it must be done every single day in order to become a habit.

Why We Fail at Creating New Habits

Most of the time, when we fail at creating a new habit, it's because we give up too easily. Things happen which throw us off our original plan and we tell ourselves that it's too hard or that we'll work on it later after circumstances change. Unexpected challenges will arise when we're trying to develop a healthy habit, just as they do in any other endeavour. That's where commitment comes into play.

The other main reason we fail at creating new habits is due to bad planning. **People decide to go too big all at once with their habit development**. Take the earlier example of developing a habit of working out daily. If you've never worked out and live a sedentary life, setting a goal of working out for an hour every day is asking for failure. The habit you're trying to develop needs to be realistic. Starting out smaller, like a 20 minute workout is much more achievable. You can always expand that once the first goal is accomplished.

Keystone Habits

In the book, The Power of Habit, author Charles Duhigg describes what he calls 'keystone habits' as habits that once people begin developing them, "they start changing other, unrelated patterns in their lives, often unknowingly." One example that he talks about in the book is that of exercise. A person begins to exercise regularly and quite often will start eating healthier and decrease unhealthy practices without even thinking about it.

The keystone habit affects many other things in a person's life, often creating a chain reaction making adding related habits more easily. This may be due in part to the natural flow of cause and effect, with the changes made influencing other areas of your life.

Another reason why a keystone habit can have such a ripple effect is that success in one area can motivate you so much that developing other healthy habits become much easier. Success tends to build upon success.

Finding Your Keystone Habit
Discovering the keystone habit or habits in your life can make the process of healthy habit creation more effective. To find your keystone habit, ask yourself these four questions and really think about the answers.

1. Which of my healthy habit goals from my plan is something I really need?

2. If this habit is established, what other areas of my life will be affected?

3. Once I change or develop this habit, will it make other changes easier?

4. Will development of this new habit be energizing and motivating to me?

Habits that fit the definition of a keystone habit will be those that produce positive answers to all four of the questions above.

Maintaining Desirable Habits
Your newly developed habits will get stronger as time goes on, but in the beginning you have to focus some effort on maintaining them. This is especially true if the new healthy habit replaced a long-term bad habit.

Maintaining desirable habits starts with the planning phase of healthy habit creation. You must choose a goal that fits your personality and lifestyle, at least to a certain degree. Trying to create a habit of something you absolutely hate to do is almost never going to be successful.

Let's go back to our earlier example of working out. If you loathe lifting weights, that would be a poor choice for creating a habit. Instead, choose something that you actually enjoy doing and it will make maintaining your habit much easier.

Once you've chosen a habit to form, continue to be specific with how you plan to accomplish the creation of the new habit. One excellent way to do this is to schedule the activity at the same time each day and make sure to clear that space on your calendar.

Saying you'll work out daily allows you to put it off until you 'have time' to do it and that usually results in procrastination and failure. Instead, set aside a specific chunk of time to accomplish that goal and stick to it.

2.2 Gamer Nutrition

While we all learned about the basics of good nutrition in high-school, it can be tough for Gamers to understand why they too need to eat a healthy, balanced diet. After all, Gamers aren't usually athletes, so why should they eat like they are training for a Marathon? Because the benefits of good nutrition go beyond achieving a ripped physique and a six-pack stomach; eating well helps to fuel your brain and your body.

Great Gamers depend on their brains, and to have a healthy brain, you need to eat a healthy diet. The type of food we eat, when we eat and how much we eat all have a huge impact on how well you can flex your cranial muscle.

Fat Can Make You Dumb

That's right folks, all that greasy pizza doesn't just make your game controller slippery, it can actually suppress your brain function. A powerful brain depends on strong blood flow throughout the body, and eating fat-filled processed foods can clog your arteries and blood vessels, restricting both oxygen and blood flow to the brain. Your brain uses blood and oxygen as food, so just like when you get famished, your brain starts to slow down - in essence, your brain power is retarded by your diet.

Sugar Weighs You Down

Just like excessive dietary fat can clog your arteries and restrict blood flow to your brain, too much sugar can have a similar effect. Eating large amounts of sugary foods like candy and sodas causes your body to act like a roller coaster - when you eat, your blood sugar spikes, giving you instant energy (and sometimes even a feeling of jitteriness or unease). That sugar high won't last though, and when you crash from it, you fall hard, feeling lethargic and unfocused. Keep up this dangerous cycle and you'll wind up overweight with type 2 diabetes, a lifelong condition that can lead to nerve damage, amputations and blindness.

Healthy Gamers Nutrition Habits

As we've already mentioned, eating a healthy balanced diet helps to control your weight, improve your reflexes and brain function, giving you the energy you need for your next marathon gaming session. As a bonus, a healthy diet can help you live a longer, healthier life.

Ready to tackle the challenge?

Here's the basics:

- ➢ **Eat a Healthy Breakfast**

  Just like mom always said, you need to start out your day with a healthy, balanced breakfast (no matter what time you roll out of bed). Breakfast is the best way to wake up your metabolism, giving your body the kick-start it needs to wake up and get moving!

- ➢ **Snack Smart**

  Limit the frequency and quantity of the snacks you eat - remember, snacks aren't meal replacements! Nosh on simple snacks like low-fat cheese sticks and unsalted nuts, apples and veggie sticks.

- ➢ **Cut Out Caffeine**

  Just like sugar, caffeine gives you an artificial high followed by a painful crash. It dehydrates you and can leave you with a splitting headache. By eliminating caffeine from your diet you will feel better and dodge the uncomfortable side effects that caffeine can have, such as excessive urination, dehydration and even diarrhoea!

- ➢ **Ditch The Sodas**

  Water should be your go-to beverage, since energy drinks, sodas and fruit juices are usually filled with empty calories that slow you down while expanding your waistline.

> ➤ **Eat Balanced Regular Meals**
>
> Mealtimes are a great excuse to take a break from the screen and spend some quality face-time with your family, friends and roomies. Aim to eat balanced meals that include lean protein, whole-grain carbs and vegetables at every meal. Resist the urge to skip meals, as this leads to wild fluctuations in your blood sugar levels and puts your metabolism on pause.

By following these simple tips, you'll be well on the way to becoming a leaner, meaner and smarter Gamer!

Body Cycle

From the moment you consume food, to the moment it is eliminated, your digestive system should be working like clockwork to eliminate what you have consumed. In order to reach peristalsis, the contraction of muscles that lead to defecation, the human body moves through the following phases:

> ➤ **Elimination (4am-12pm)**
>
> **Breakfast**
>
> During this period, your body is still trying to eliminate what you have eaten the day before. For breakfast, make sure you have a light meal and up until lunch have healthy snacks it needed.

> ➤ **Food Intake (12pm-8pm)**
>
> **Lunch till Dinner**
>
> During this period, you should focus on eating meals that are made of at least 75% Vegetables and/or Salad. Always drink a glass of water first, as well as a side salad; this will aid digestion. If you want to snack, focus on nuts that contain healthy fats -- like Brazil nuts -- and fruit.

➢ **Digestion (8pm-4am)**

Sleep (and Gaming)

It is during the digestive period that your body will process everything you have eaten during the course of the day. This task involves breaking down food into molecules, absorbing nutrients, and preparing for elimination. It is a good idea to stop eating after 8pm in order to allow this process to continue. However, if you feel hungry, you could try drinking herbal tea, or water. If necessary, eat fruit.

Remember that lack of sleep can cause you to eat more with more food your body needs to work harder, meaning less energy for you and this can make you sluggish.

2.3 Avatar Health

Your body or your "Life Avatar" controls your "Game Avatar". Meaning your mind and body are all part of the gaming experience, therefore you need both of these to be efficient and effective for an enhanced and healthy gaming experience.

➢ **Fitness**

Aerobic exercise such as jogging is a key component for weight loss and building endurance. To receive the optimal health benefits, it is important to increase your normal heart rate for at least thirty minutes per workout. Jogging or brisk walking requires little in the way of equipment, all you really need is a heart rate monitor and a good pair of running shoes.

➢ **Posture (Core Strength)**

Regular gaming can be rough on your posture, which in turn can cause pain and discomfort. The Vitality Challenge acknowledges that a great way to combat this is with the practice of Yoga and Pilates which not only strengthens your core, but is also beneficial for relaxation and stress relief.

> **Eyesight**

We've established that prolonged game play can cause eye strain and fatigue. A few preventative measures that can be taken to diminish these issues include ensuring the contrast and brightness of your gaming screen is set properly and avoiding glare. It's also advisable to take frequent breaks to change your visual focal point, as these steps can go a long way in preventing eye strain problems in the first place. There are also Eye Exercises you can do to which will help most people keep their eyes efficient.

2.4 Gamer Rage Reduction

As a Gamer you will be familiar with the fact that mild stress can often turn to 'Gamer Rage'. Whether it comes as a result of other platform players, or your own performance, Gamer Rage can leave you unhappy and unable to play. Fortunately, it is possible to both solve and prevent Gamer Rage through relaxation techniques such as focused breathing techniques.

> **Focused Breathing Techniques**

Since the early 12th century, both men and women in the Middle East have practiced Hatha yoga. Their main motivation for doing this was to improve their ability to deal with life's major stresses, as well as adopting ways to deal with stress as it approaches. To see the benefits of Hatha yoga, you do not need to become a full devotee. Each time you experience stress as a result of a game you are playing, you should breathe in for seven seconds, and exhale for the same period of time. By doing this, your stress levels will lower, and in future you will be less likely to experience Gamer Rage.

➢ **Clear Breaks**

Do not use Gaming as pure stress relief or bring external frustrations into your gaming sessions. Clear your mind before a gaming session, this can be done by either using a focused breathing technique or by releasing stress through exercise or even a 30 minute walk. If you don't have the time or patience for 30 minutes, at least take 5 minutes out to clear your head, do some eye exercises or stretches before you start. Just make sure you have a routine and stick by it.

➢ **Reduce Sugary and Fatty Food**

High in sugar foods and drinks will give you energy highs, although they will also later give you an energy low. Also, fatty foods can make you sluggish and lethargic; both the Sugar and Fatty consumables can cause irritability, which leads to enhanced Gamer Rage. If you want to avoid it and keep a cool winning head, eat healthy.

2.5 Weight Loss

Weight Loss is only good when it is healthy and is sustainable long-term. The creation of beneficial habits is key to a healthy lifestyle and key to creating sustainable weight loss.

Following these key habits for optimal weight loss:

➢ **Burn more calories**

One of the key factors to weight loss is to burn more calories than you consume. Of course you might say! Although, doing 30 minutes exercise a day is great, you need to burn calories many times during the day. Add more physical activity to your day; move more; do not go for convenience, aim for inconvenience that works out that body of yours (ie. walk instead of drive). Don't Sleep, Eat and Game in the same room.

➤ **Fat Burning Jog (Exercise)**

Show the world you are alive by moving that body. Jogging and walking are great for general fitness and assisting with weight loss. The most important thing is taking action, as you will not lose weight by talking about it.

➤ **Good Nutrition**

Different body types and cultures eat differently, but as a rule of thumb the body needs nutrition from a variety of sources such as fruit, vegetables, seeds and beans.

➤ **Drink Water**

Water is one of the key ingredients your body needs to lose weight and keep it off. A decrease in water intake will increase fat deposits, so ensure you're eating habits include water rich foods and healthy water consumption. Also, hunger can mimic thrust, meaning if you feel hungry you could just be thirsty, so have a glass of water prior to eating.

➤ **Sleep**

Your body needs to rest, even though you might not want to. Sleep researchers have found that a lack of sleep impacts your health, safety, and longevity. So, ensure you receive 7 to 9 hours of sleep each day.

The "Sleep Medicine Program" at the New York University School of Medicine in New York City has found that when you don't get enough sleep, there is a chance you will not feel as satisfied after you eat. Also, lack of sleep can stimulate your appetite, meaning you want to eat more. This combination means you will have a higher chance of over eating when you have lack of sleep.

2.6 Kid Gamers

The technological advancement of today makes it inevitable for kids to take up computer gaming. While it only took a few hours of children's weekly average play a decade ago, computer gaming is the major form of play for the kids of today. Accessibility of electronic gadgets and busier parents can be attributed to the decreasing trend of the energetic, lively and healthy physical form of play.

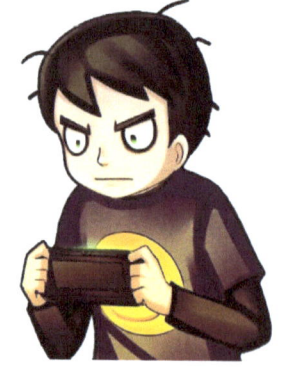

It is therefore imperative for parents to teach their children good computer gaming habits. You can still raise healthy kids without taking them away from their computer games. One good way is to design a point system that would allow a certain amount of playing time. You can give them points for good deeds like cleaning their room, playing outside or taking the dog for a walk. Healthy habits like eating fruits and vegetables and taking up a sport can also merit them point. While unhealthy activities will mean demerits.

"This will assist with healthy habit creation for your children."

Here is an example of a point system, Activities:

- ➢ Make the bed (5 Points)
- ➢ Clean the room (10 Points)
- ➢ Eat your Vegetables (25 points)
- ➢ 30 Minute Jog (50 Points)
- ➢ Train for a sport (65 Points)
- ➢ Took out the trash (50 Points)
- ➢ Make Bed every day for a week (50 points)
- ➢ Drink soft drink (-10 points)
- ➢ Drink Energy Drink (-25 points)

Gaming Time
100 points allows one hour gaming time. Additional 15 minutes will be added if playing with another member of the family. No gaming before homework is done.

The idea is to have the points allocated to the areas you want your child to create healthy habits like eating healthy foods, taking up sports and being an active and helpful member of the family. Children that do sports training actually create habits that develop self-discipline.

Self-discipline is important as they grow older and more independent. Another important factor is parent participation. Take an active role in your kids' activities. This will not only help you monitor their activities - gaming can also be a great bonding time for you and your child, one that they will appreciate even after they have long grown out of computer games.

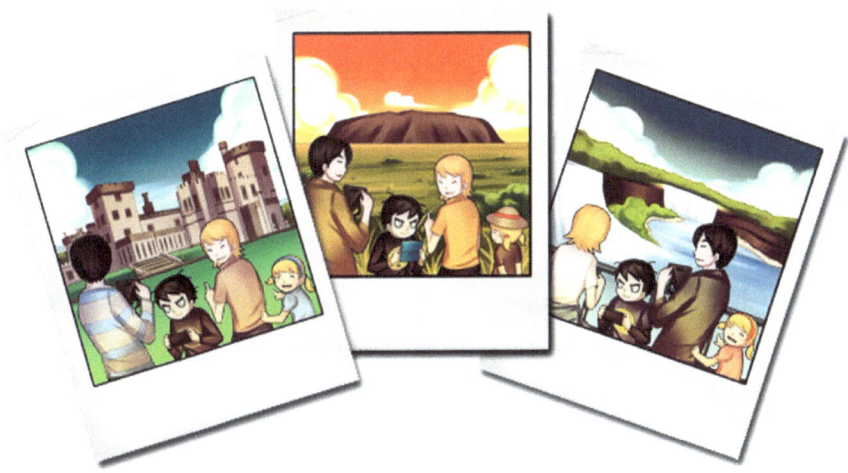

3. Vitality Challenge

The Vitality Challenge teaches healthier living for vitality gaming, through the creation of healthy habits.

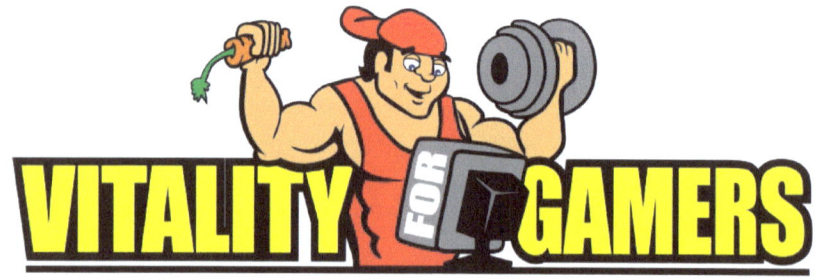

"Creating healthy habits is key,
although start with 2 habits to begin with.
Trying to do everything, you will end up doing nothing."

To Do:
- ➢ Select 1 or 2 Habits from the Vitality Challenge
- ➢ Write down the Habits and goals you want to achieve
- ➢ Put this where you will see it every day
- ➢ Share with someone (make yourself accountable)
- ➢ Commit to the habit/s for at least 30 days (90 days preferred)
- ➢ Once you create the habit/s, select more habits gradually

3.1 Breakfast

Throughout the typical day of a Gamer, the human body goes through Cycles: food ingestion, food digestion, and elimination. Each stage of this day involves a different part of the digestive system, which will be working continuously to process nutrients and maintain optimal health. In order to achieve peak health, Gamers should make themselves aware of these cycles, what they involve, and how they can aid them by eating the correct foods. While certain foods provide the nutrients needed for good health and fast digestion, others will clog up the digestive system, leading to feelings like fatigue and sluggishness.

From the moment you consume food, to the moment it is eliminated, your digestive system should be working like clockwork to eliminate what you have consumed.

Fruit for Breakfast
When you are eating your breakfast, your digestive system is working through the elimination stage. Focusing on fruit will keep it light enough to not disrupt this process, and it will ensure you receive the nutrients you need for both short and long term health. A fruit only breakfast will provide you with vitamins, antioxidants, and fluids. Focus on choosing at least one energy rich food, such as bananas which are vital for mental and physical stimulation. Eating a fruit only breakfast will get you through to lunchtime.

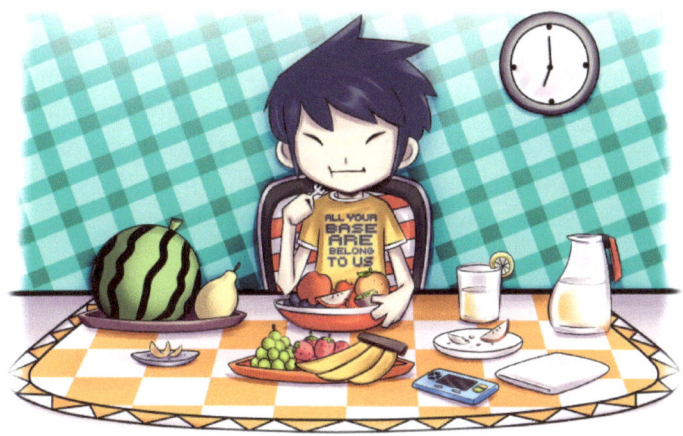

Creating the right fruit only breakfast
As well as adding the energy rich foods mentioned before, you should try to vary the colors used. By using at least three different colors, you will stand a stronger chance of achieving the blend of vitamins needed to support your body throughout the day.

Foods to avoid
Try to avoid consuming anything that is binding or too heavy. Eggs are often promoted as a great food for breakfast, but they can lead to constipation and will therefore disrupt the digestive process. Foods like cereal and toast can cause bloating and gas. Not only does this make gamers feel uncomfortable, it also impedes the digestive process. Finally, some cereals can cause mid-morning energy crashes.

3.2 Gamer Snacks

Although gaming is a relatively sedentary activity in terms of physical exertion, it is one that can drain your energy in surprising amounts. A typical gamer will experience fatigue as a result of concentration, as well as consistent movements. Of course, this depends on the game being played and the console, but each Gamer does need a litany of healthy snacks and habits to get them through a long session nonetheless.

The need for healthy snacks while gaming
Anyone who has considered themselves to be a Gamer for any length of time will tell you that the temptation to snack while playing is almost unbearable. Snacking is often associated with weight gain, but that does not have to be the case. By focusing on snacks that are healthy, tasty, and filling, it is possible to sustain yourself, meet the needs of your cravings, and prevent weight gain at the same time.

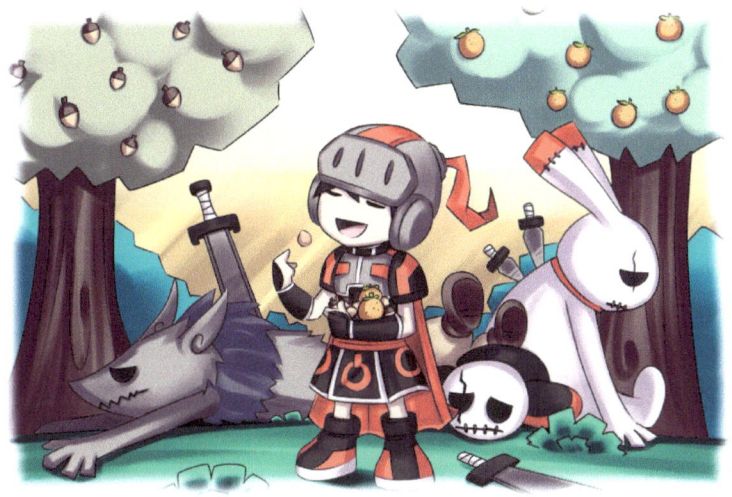

The case for focusing on healthy snacks grows stronger when you consider the impact that sugary foods have on your energy levels. Although, you may experience a peak initially, once your body has had time to process what you have eaten, you will crash. This leads to fatigue, irritability, and poor concentration. If you want to be at the top of your game, as well as healthy, you will choose diet-friendly snacks over their sugary counterparts each time.

One very troublesome side effect that is overlooked when considering the benefits of healthy snacks over junk food is Gamer Rage. While it is inevitable that each game player will experience this at some point during the course of their life, it becomes more frequent when you fail to eat nutritiously. The energy highs and lows mentioned above are associated with irritability, which leads to enhanced Gamer Rage. If you want to avoid it and keep a cool winning head, eat healthy snacks.

Choosing the right snack selection

Contrary to popular belief, healthy snacking is not time consuming, or boring. There are plenty of healthy foods out there that taste great, you just need a little education before finding them. First of all, you should turn to water or herbal tea when you experience hunger pangs. Thirst can often mask itself as hunger, so hydrating before assuming you need to eat is wise. Next, you should focus on achieving a mix of healthy fats, proteins, and energy boosting foods. Brazil nuts provide energy in the form of healthy fats and proteins, while bananas will sustain your mental alertness and physical energy for far longer than many other snacks. These foods don't have to be eaten plain either; take almonds soaked in water with sprinkled cinnamon: they will boost your energy levels and support your body in remaining healthy at the same time.

Healthy Snack Examples

- ➢ **Pop Corn**

  Not only is popcorn cheap and easy to make, it is relatively low in calories when you take the salted option, it will help you feel fuller for longer, and it will give you a stable energy boost. Do bear in mind that eating salted popcorn can dehydrate you, and make a conscious effort to remain hydrated.

- ➢ **Nachos and cheese**

  Despite being associated with high calories, nachos and cheese can fast become a healthy gamer snack. Choose low calorie, low salt tortillas, and top them with low-fat mozzarella. This incredibly moreish snack is filling and healthy.

➢ **Nuts**

Purchase a few mixed nut packs before you embark on an all-night gaming session, and you will be able to fill yourself with several food groups and nutrients that will help you make it through the night. Nuts are rich in healthy fats, proteins, and some carbohydrates. The balance they provide will provide you with energy and overall vitality.

Also, try soaking your Nuts.

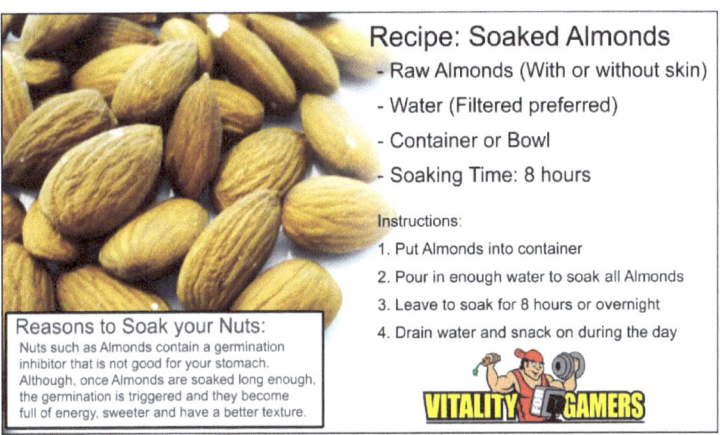

Recipe: Soaked Almonds
- Raw Almonds (With or without skin)
- Water (Filtered preferred)
- Container or Bowl
- Soaking Time: 8 hours

Instructions:
1. Put Almonds into container
2. Pour in enough water to soak all Almonds
3. Leave to soak for 8 hours or overnight
4. Drain water and snack on during the day

Reasons to Soak your Nuts:
Nuts such as Almonds contain a germination inhibitor that is not good for your stomach. Although, once Almonds are soaked long enough, the germination is triggered and they become full of energy, sweeter and have a better texture.

VITALITY GAMERS

➢ **Hummus**

Whether it is home-made or store bought, hummus is a healthy and filling snack that is ideal for all night gaming. If you want to make it yourself, you simply need to blend a can of chickpeas with two tablespoons of olive oil. To jazz it up a little, you can mix it with a variety of ingredients, like chillies, black pepper, or lemon. Eat it with crackers or sliced vegetables, and keep it by your side while you game.

➢ **Fruit and vegetables**

In terms of providing energy and nutrients at the same time, fruit and vegetables are no-brainers. Many gamers are put off by the idea that they are dull, but that is not the case. A vibrant fruit salad with a little honey on top is as sweet as any candy, and it won't cause you to experience the energy crashes and gamer rage associated with eating food laced with synthetic sugar.

➢ **Crusty wholegrain bread**

We all know that carbohydrates are great in terms of providing energy, but very few people head for the right ones when they want to make their way through an all-night gaming session. Wholegrain carbohydrates are better for your digestive system, and will provide slow burning energy. You can add a little low-fat spread to make it tastier, or even some cream cheese.

➢ **Feta cheese**

Feta cheese is typically used in Greek salads, but tastes great by itself too. You could toast it with some pita bread, or even eat it by itself.

➢ **Salsa**

Whether you buy ready-made salsa or make it at home, it can act as a great additive to toasted pita bread and chopped vegetables. As a healthy, tasty, and easy snack, salsa is addictive without being bad for you.

➢ **Sushi**

Finally, if you want a snack that is a little more luxurious, try sushi. It is a little challenging to make, but many stores now sell it pre-made, or you can even get Japanese takeout. If you are not a fish fan, try chicken, vegetables, or duck instead.

3.3 Meals

Gamers need fuel. The human body consumes calories even while at rest. So if you are sitting for an all-night gaming session, you still need good food to fuel your body. The fuel of choice for many Gamers happens to be junk food. How often have you heard your friends talking about a late night run for soda and tortilla chips? While there is nothing wrong with having junk food on occasion, fuelling your body with junk constantly is a very bad habit to have.

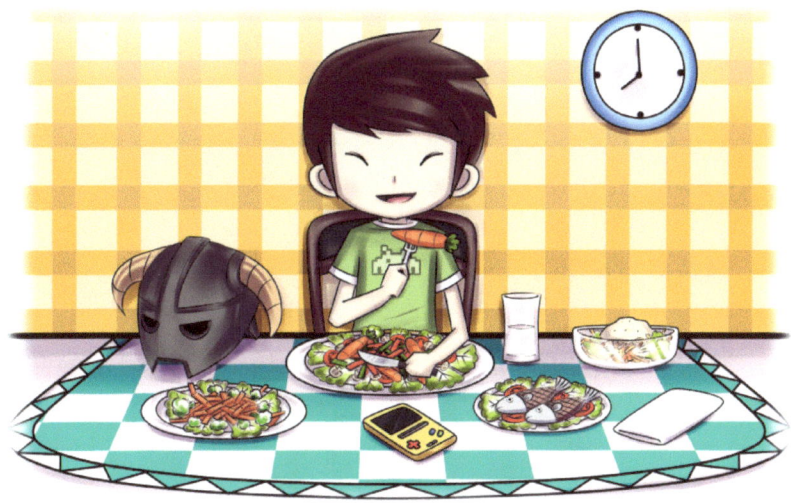

Poor eating habits lead to poor nutrition. You must have the proper amount of vitamins and nutrients supplied to your body in order for it to function. While this might sound like something your grade school physical education teacher said, it's true. To put this in perspective: good nutrition can help your gaming performance. The right balance of nutrients will improve your eye/hand co-ordination, increase reaction speed, and help you make complex decisions.

"In other words, eat well if you want to beat that boss."

Benefits of Healthy Eating

A balanced diet is what helps you get the good nutrition we just talked about. It isn't about how many pizza slices you can balance on your plate, either. Diets that are balanced have the right amount of each type of food needed to supply different nutrients.

A good rule of thumb when trying to create a balanced diet is to 'eat a rainbow'. What we mean is to eat fruits and vegetables that are richly colored. Rich, deep colors indicate different benefits when it comes to essential vitamins.

➢ **Red**

Fruits and vegetables that are red colored are a source of lycopene. This antioxidant performs important tasks by helping to prevent or repair cell damage in the body.

➢ **Yellow/Orange**

Chock-full of Vitamin A. This vitamin also helps fight against cell damage. Yellow/orange foods also help with eye disorders and improve vision.

➢ **Purple/blue**

Another powerhouse of antioxidants. Eating foods that are blue or purple improve memory and other brain functions.

➢ **Green**

Leafy green vegetables have B vitamins and some contain lutein. Again, more vitamins and nutrients to help the eyes. B vitamins are known to increase energy.

➢ **White**

Certain white vegetables and fruits contain the chemical allicin. This chemical helps reduce blood pressure which is important for people that may experience 'Gamer Rage'.

Eat Less Red Meat

Eating too much red meat can lead to high cholesterol levels which in turn put one at higher risk for heart attack and stroke. Red meat isn't bad if consumed in lesser quantities than other meats. A 20 year study conducted by Harvard University found that people who eat less red meat live longer than people who eat a lot of red meat. Just cutting your consumption of red meat (like beef) to once a week or less can add years to your life. That adds up to extra gaming years!

Try replacing the red meat you consume with another meat you enjoy – fish or chicken. Remember to limit your intake of pork, it has a high salt content. Other high protein foods can be substituted. Try beans, nuts, and tofu. You might think tofu is gross, but try marinating it before cooking. Tofu takes on the favor of the marinade or the food it is cooked with.

Eat Fish (Omega 3 and health benefits)

While cutting red meat consumption, replace the meat with a fish of your choice. Fish, especially wild ocean fish, are full of Omega 3 fatty acids. This fat is hard to find from other foods, and is hard to absorb from certain non-manufactured sources. For example, some grains contain Omega 3s, but to gain access to the fatty acids you must grind them at home or the Omega 3s will lose potency.

Omega 3 fatty acids have documented health benefits. Joint health, eye health, brain function, and even lowering cholesterol have all been proven by scientific studies. In fact, fish oil and Omega 3s are so good for your health supplements have been created from ultra-concentrated fish oil!

3.4 Fitness

As the number of people who play video games increases, so do the concern of health experts about the effects of gaming on physical fitness. Since 2008, the number of people who claim to play video games has risen 241% in the USA. As the rate of obesity increases among adolescents and young adults, many health experts have questioned the role of gaming in weight gain. Some studies have shown correlation between gaming and increased caloric intake, while others suggest the sedentary nature of gaming has contributed to the obesity epidemic.

"Some studies suggest that a sedentary lifestyle can be just as damaging as smoking to one's health."

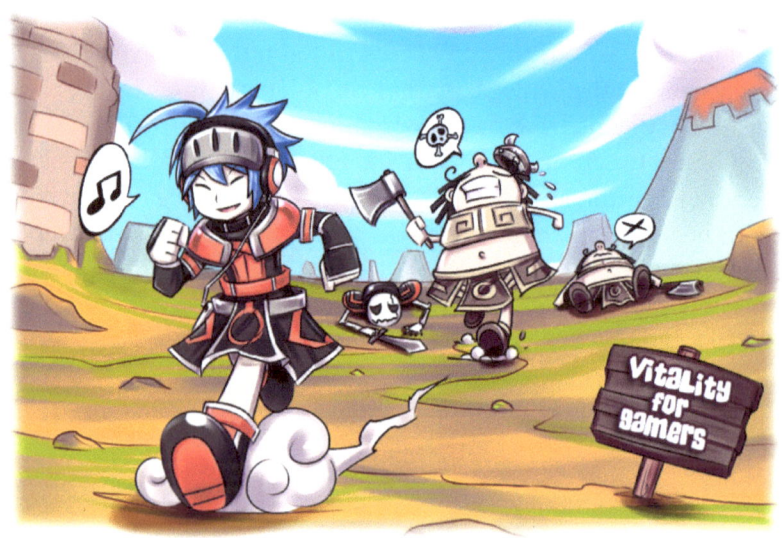

Pre-game Preparations

Your body is the medium in which you play games; without an effective and efficient body you are not playing at your peak and the impact of long gaming sessions on your body is so much higher. Treat your body well and obtain fitness for enhanced gaming and longevity.

➢ Full Meal

Many Gamers will play till all hours of the night and some even spend days on extended gaming, taking only brief snack breaks. Thus, it is recommended getting a full stomach as part of pre-game preparation.

Eat Healthy - Eating a healthy balanced meal containing of at least 75% vegetables will give you a steady flow of energy, in combination with healthy snacks and water.

Avoid high fat or greasy foods – These foods will make you sluggish and slow.

Avoid high Sugary foods – You will have a high energy burst with an eventually deep low. You will find yourself continually needing high sugary foods to boost your performance.

➢ Clear Break

Do not use Gaming as pure stress relief or bring external frustrations into your gaming sessions. Clear your mind before a gaming session, this can be done by either using a focused breathing technique or by releasing stress through exercise or even a 30 minute walk. If you don't have the time or patience for 30 minutes, at least take 5 minutes out to clear your head, do some eye exercises or stretches before you start. Just make sure you have a routine and stick by it.

➢ Exercise

Just like with anything else, a person needs to be physically fit to optimally perform when gaming. Physical exercise, especially done right before sitting down for a session of gaming, can increase the blood flow to the brain, which helps concentration and reaction time. Additionally, physical exercise increases the strength of bones and muscles, which can help prevent repetitive stress injuries and circulation issues associated with prolonged periods of sitting.

Getting into an exercise routine will benefit you in both gaming and your real world life. Here are some pre-game exercises that can help getting your body active and alert for the games;

Walking - This is the most natural form of exercise. Take a 30 minute walk and get a nice leg stretching stroll. If you don't feel like going out, there are also activities you can do at home that can serve the purpose. You can make dinner, clean up, do some gardening or a hobby that requires you to move around and not sit.

Jogging - For a more energetic choice, jogging will not only have your blood running, a jog as short as 30 minutes can also burn off some of those stored fat. If you can't go outside for a jog; spend an hour cleaning the house or a hobby that requires you to move around and not sit.

Fat Burning Jog - The fat burning jog will increase gamer endurance and help with weight loss. The aim is not to jog until you drop; it is to increase your heart rate to an optimal fat burning rate for at least 30 minutes.

There are numerous ways to calculate this rate and the following is just one of them. Start jogging (or even walking), plan a routine and then settle into a rate that is comfortable for you.

You will need a heart rate monitor to keep track of your heart rate. A basic setup watch and chest strap product will work fine. These can be found in most sports stores.

Casual Challenge *(Unfit or new to jogging)*
Heart rate range:
(**170 minus** your Age) to (**180 minus** your Age)

Active Challenge (Generally fit)
Heart rate range:
(**175 minus** your Age) to (**185 minus** your Age)

Hardcore Challenge (Exercise regularly)
Heart rate range:
(**180 minus** your Age) to (**190 minus** your Age)

Push-ups and Crunches - These exercises are ideal while you wait for the applications to load or while you're setting up your equipment. You can also do sets of push-ups or crunches while your system is re-spawning.

Exercises and Stretches during Games

It is also advised that you incorporate stretching and walking into the long hours of gaming. Take advantage of loading and re-spawning time to take short walks while stretching. In fact, you can more than just walking. Hype yourself up with a Dance, Push-Ups or Acting Out. These respites from sedentary sitting can increase the flow of blood to your brain, invigorating focus, attention and body reaction.
(See: Quick Guides – Gamer Stretches)

Sit-Stand Desks

Some Gamers are opting to use sit stand desks for many reasons. The adjustable desks can be used while the user is sitting and can be adjusted to a height where the user can play comfortably while standing. This is a good choice of desks for hard core Gamers. The standing position can give them more flexibility and at the same time relieves them from the cramps of sitting too long. Additionally, playing while standing will allow Gamers to increase movement of their bodies more, allowing them to burn calories as they play.

Exercises and Stretches

Here are some easy to do yet effective exercise routines that you can do while in the game;

> *Stretches* - Occasionally do the stretching while you are at play. You can concentrate on one particular part of your body at a time. Start with neck stretching, arms, upper body and then leg stretching. Walking for a minute or two can also help you relax from the strain.

> *Eye Exercises* - A series of eye exercises done from time to time during the game will relieve strain to your eyes.

> *Wrist Exercises* - Avoid long continuous typing or wrist use. This will strain your wrists and will eventually lead to more serious problems including carpal tunnel syndrome. Make sure to take frequent breaks from wrist use. Also, do quick and effective wrist exercises to relieve the strain. One simple wrist exercise is simply shaking your hands.

Freely shaking the hands for a minute will encourage blood to flow back to your hands. Making fists for at least 10 seconds and then relaxing is another good routine. Do as many intervals as you can while you wait for your game applications to re-load or re-spawn.

➢ *Head Rolls* - This exercise is effective in reducing neck, shoulder, head and eye tension. Start the exercise by sitting straight, closing your eyes and dropping your head forward. Take a deep breath and relax your shoulders, and then slowly rotate your head towards one side, back, the other side and then back to the front. Keep your shoulders steady and relaxed while you rotate your head.

3.5 Drink

As one of the most vital dietary components needed to ensure good human health, water needs to be consumed frequently and consciously. Our bodies are made up of 60% water, it is central to various life processes, and provides positive side effects like clear skin and aiding weight loss. Despite water being so beneficial, many people fail to consume the recommended 6-8 glasses per day. By failing to do this, they are preventing their bodies from functioning at optimal levels.

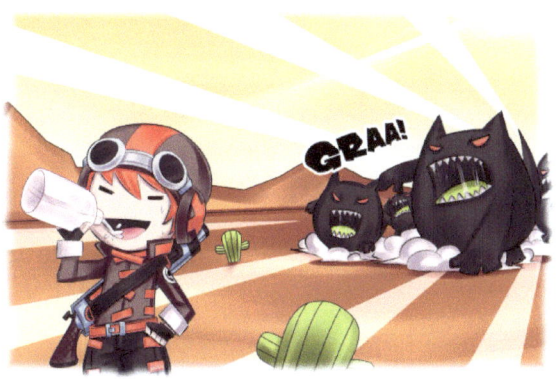

Consuming more water
One of the main reasons people fail to drink 6-8 glasses per day is that doing so can be quite inconvenient. If you work, have children, or fall prey to a million other distractions, your mind is less likely to jump to hydration. One of the easiest ways to consume more water is to invest in a 1 litre re-useable flask, fill it, and carry it around with you. You will soon find that you consume more water than usual. In addition to this, you should focus your diet on water-rich foods. Try eating a side of salad with your lunch and dinner, and fill it with cucumber, lettuce, and celery. Finally, if you feel hungry, drink water rather than eating a snack. Thirst often mimics hunger, which means you could be hydrating yourself while promoting weight loss.

Water for vitality
By consuming plenty of water each day, you will be supporting several body organs in their vital life processes. By staying well-hydrated, you will aid your vascular system in delivering nutrients and oxygen to the cells in your body. Drinking a steady amount of water provides more fluids for such nutrients to diffuse through when they are trying to reach tissues. Drinking plenty of water is also one of the best ways to prevent constipation; the more you consume, the softer your stools will be. Water will ultimately lubricate your joints; for gamers this is essential -- as sitting in one position for a long period of time can lead to joint stiffness. Finally, the molecular construction of water means it can help regulate your body temperature. Again, when sitting in the same position for a long period of time, achieving body temperature regulation can be difficult. Hydration can provide you with overall physical comfort.

Water for weight loss
While scientists have long suspected that drinking plenty of water can lead to weight loss, it has only been in recent years that solid evidence has emerged to back this theory up. In a large-scale study conducted at Virginia Tech, it was found that those who actively consume 2-3 glasses of water prior to eating a meal will lose weight. For those who leave a sedentary to moderately active lifestyle, this is great news in terms of weight loss and overall health.

Water for great skin

Although some scientists believe that water's contribution to clear skin is open to debate, there is evidence to show that extra consumption reduces the likelihood of developing or sustaining conditions like acne. Drinking around 500ml of water naturally increases blood flow to your skin; this in turn creates a healthy glow. In addition to this, water's impact on general health can lead to a reduction in the bacteria that gather and cause poor skin.

By making a conscious effort to drink more water, you can enhance your overall health and appearance. In addition to this, you will feel more comfortable while gaming.

3.6 Posture

Modern technology has brought the consumer many fun and exciting digital experiences including video games. As with all good things there is often a downside or risk involved. In the case of long extended periods of sitting, as is so typical during the activity of video gaming there are risks to general health and posture in specific. Maintaining or improving good posture after long periods of sitting, especially while in front of a computer or TV screen, is critical to wellness and good health. Fortunately there are a number of techniques and exercises, as well as specially designed desks that can improve and help to maintain better posture.

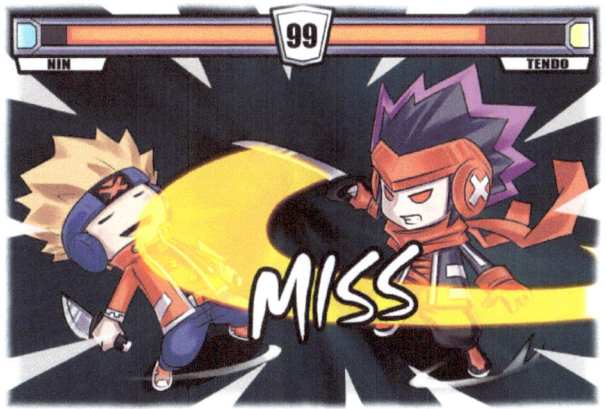

Poor Posture can Ultimately Lead to Chronic Back Pain

Most medical professionals will agree that maintaining poor posture for long periods of time can lead to spinal problems and other skeletal and muscular injuries. In addition, maintaining the wrong posture while both sitting and standing or lying down can ultimately lead to chronic back pain. One of the simplest and easiest ways to address poor posture is through changing the way you sit. This can be accomplished by first ensuring that the feet are always firmly and flatly on the floor. It is also important to ensure that the thighs maintain a parallel position with regard to the floor, as well as the hips and knees being parallel. In addition, the shoulders should be in a loose and relaxed state, while the forearms are maintained in relatively parallel alignment with the floor.

Yoga and Pilates

Along with the proper sitting posture described, it is also important to avoid leaning back in a chair as this can strain the neck and pull on back muscles, ultimately leading to further chronic back pain. Certain core strengthening exercises such as Yoga and Pilates can also improve one's posture and overall skeletal and muscular strength. By participating in activities like Yoga and Pilates, an individual is far more likely to offset the negative effects of long hours of sitting. In the case of video games, gamer posture is especially important due to the extraordinarily long hours of sitting that are typically involved in this type of activity. Other factors can also aggravate poor posture such as being overweight or obese or being exposed to excessive levels of stress.

The Sit-Stand Desk

Finally, another excellent tool for improving one's posture is the sit-stand desk. The sit-stand desk is essentially an ergonomically designed desk that is intended to improve or maintain an individual's healthy posture. These innovative and effective desks are offered in manual and electric versions. In either version, the working surface of the desk is adjusted to comfortable levels throughout the day. These desks are designed to improve the comfort level of those who spend long hours sitting and working in front a video screen. In the case of gamer posture, these desks are quite useful in reducing the strains and stresses of long hours of sitting. In summary, it can be said that good gamer posture is easy to achieve and is vitally important to one's long-term physical health.

3.7 Oxygen

When it comes to improving your overall health and reducing the stress experienced when gaming, many players do not realize that paying a little extra attention to their breathing rate could go a long way. In recent years a growing body of evidence has begun to demonstrate that well-focused and paced breathing can reduce stress, promote overall long-term health, and improve performance in terms of concentration. In addition to this, the nature of gaming means that those who dedicate their spare time to their favorite game need to pay more attention than others to how they breathe. Fortunately, it is possible to improve your breathing and therefore your overall health by dedicating just a few minutes a day to deep breathing practices.

Gamer Health

As any devoted player will know, the art of gaming can often become quite stressful. With stress comes several short and long-term side-effects. For example, in the short-term you can easily develop conditions such as hypertension, aka high blood pressure. In the long-term, such conditions can lead to you developing other forms of heart disease. Fortunately, recent research has demonstrated that people who choose to spend at least five to ten minutes a day practicing deep breathing techniques can regulate their blood pressure. As a gamer, you will spend the majority of your day engaging in shallow breathing techniques. This means that your heart has to spend more time pumping hard to compensate for the lack of oxygen you take in with your short breaths. While it is not possible to consciously engage in deep breathing throughout all your waking hours, taking a few moments on a daily basis can help you give your heart a rest, and it can also lead to naturally slower breathing practices. In the short-term, this means that you will have lower blood pressure. In the long-term, you are less likely to experience adverse coronary events like angina or a heart attack.

When it comes to reducing stress, the benefits you will experience will extend far beyond your heart. As a gamer you need your mental health to be in check too, and by using breathing techniques to reduce your stress levels you can achieve that. Next time you find yourself feeling angry because of gaming challenges, take a minute or two to breathe in deeply. By doing this, you are more likely to adopt a happy frame of mind. In turn, this happy frame of mind will enhance your ability to concentrate, which will place you at the top of your game.

Gamer Rage

As a gamer you will be familiar with the fact that mild stress can often turn to gamer rage. Whether it comes as a result of other platform players, or your own performance, gamer rage can leave you unhappy and unable to play. Fortunately, it is possible to both solve and prevent gamer rage through the use of focused breathing techniques. Since the early 12th century, both men and women in the Middle East have practiced Hatha yoga. Their main motivation for doing this was to improve their ability to deal with life's major stresses, as well as adopting ways to deal with stress as it approaches. To see the benefits of Hatha yoga, you do not need to become a full devotee. Each time you experience stress as a result of a game you are playing, you should breathe in for seven seconds, and exhale for the same period of time. By doing this, your stress levels will lower, and in future you will be less likely to experience gamer rage.

Vitality Breath

If you would like to place yourself on the right track when it comes to improving your breathing, gaming techniques, and overall health, you should consider the "Vitality Breath". With this breath you can improve the functioning of your lymphatic system. As the system that supports your immunological defenses, the lymphatic system undergoes a lot of stress. (See: Quick Guides – Vitality Breath)

Vitality Breath:
- ➢ Breath In for a ratio of 1
- ➢ Hold your Breath for a ratio of 4
- ➢ Breath out for a ratio of 2
- ➢ Repeat the above steps 5 times, daily

As an example, if you breathe in for 5 seconds, you would hold your breath for 20 seconds and then breathe out for 10 seconds. Make sure you are relaxed during this and as you improve, increase the amount of time from 5 seconds.

Make sure you always breathe at a pace you are comfortable with, if you are straining to hold your breath, then reduce the number of seconds.

This is something that can easily be done wherever you are, and it takes no time at all to do. For the best gaming experience do this prior to Gaming sessions and also once during gaming breaks.

By taking a few minutes out of your daily routine, you can seriously enhance your health as well as your gaming techniques. Well-focused breathing is not just needed for great cardiovascular, mental, and lymphatic health; it can help with many areas of your body. As scientists have recently discovered that better breathing leads to less waste and therefore healthier kidneys, it is clear that the benefits of deep breathing and other techniques cannot be understated. To see your health improve drastically, get stuck in to conscious breathing techniques today.

3.8 Eye Sight

Ask any gamer which of their 5 senses is most important to them, and the hands-down answer will be their eyesight. Gamers rely on healthy eyesight to play virtually all computer games.

How Extended Screen-time Can Hurt (Your Eyes)
Whether you're a hardcore gamer, an Internet junkie or a movie buff, spending hours in front of a computer monitor or TV screen can wreak havoc on your eyesight. If you've experienced eyestrain, dry eyes, fuzzy vision, headaches and/or neck and upper shoulder pain while gaming, chances are good you might have Computer Vision Syndrome (CVS).

According to the American Optometric Association, the frequency and severity of CVS symptoms is directly related to screen time duration - the longer you spend gaming, the more severe the symptoms. Pre-existing vision problems like astigmatism, poor eye coordination or age-related vision loss can all aggravate the symptoms of CVS.

Gaming-related vision problems develop because looking at a screen is hard work (for your eyes, that is). Your eyes have to fight to focus in on the rapid movements while combatting the glare and unnaturally close viewing angles - let's face it, with the exception of a TV or computer screen, you don't usually spend hours staring at something that's less than a few feet away from you, right?

Ironically, gaming can also lead to weakening of the eye muscles. How so? Because your eyes aren't designed to focus on a fixed location for hours on end. Doing so can cause the muscles around your eyes to become fatigued, leading to blurry vision.

Want to protect your eyesight from the dangers of the screen? Read on for some great tips and tricks on how to not only preserve your vision, but maybe even enhance it!

Don't Forget to Blink
It might sound obvious, but one of the leading causes of eye strain for gamers is caused by vision fixation - a common occurrence for all screen users. Ever watch a little kid watching TV? They don't blink, and chances are, you don't either. Make a conscious effort to blink while gaming. This will help prevent dry eyes, the leading cause of eye strain and soreness.

Hey You, Look Over Here!
To prevent the negative effects of screen fixation, regularly look away from the monitor, focusing your eyes on an object that is 10-20 feet away. Doing this every 15-20 minutes while gaming will allow your eyes to refocus, helping to minimize eyestrain.

Step Away From The Screen
While brief 'refocus breaks' are a great way to temporarily relieve eyestrain, during marathon gaming sessions your whole body needs a break. For every hour you spend gaming, plan on taking a 10-15 minute break where you get up and walk around. This will help relax your eyes and give you time to attend to other pressing needs, like eating and going to the bathroom.

Eating For Eyesight
Healthy eyes rely on a healthy diet. Lutein and zeaxanthin are two naturally-occurring substances that have been positively linked to better eyesight. Researchers believe that these substances help to prevent harmful blue light from reaching the back of the eye and damaging the retina, acting as a type of 'edible sunglasses'. Zeaxanthin and lutein occur naturally in many fruits and veggies, including:

- Mangos
- Broccoli
- Oranges
- Peaches
- Dark lettuce
- Limit your Sugar intake

Protecting your vision also means limiting your intake of refined sugars. Obesity and excessive consumption of refined sugars is one of the leading causes of adult-onset (type 2) diabetes, the leading cause of vision loss in America today. Consider cutting down on (or even eliminating) sodas, sweets and processed foods from your diet - your eyes, and your waistline, will thank you.

3.8.1 Eye Breaks

Give your eyes frequent breaks with the following techniques for eyesight longevity. (See: Quick Guides – Vitality Vision)

➢ **Blinking**

Make a conscious effort to blink on occasion while gaming. ***Benefit:*** *One of the leading causes of eye strain for gamers is caused by vision fixation, blinking helps with this.*

➢ **Focus Break**

While gaming take a few second breaks every 5 - 10 minutes and focus on an object around the room, choose a different object each time. If playing for over an hour, get up and walk around. ***Benefit:*** *One of the leading causes of eye strain for gamers is caused by vision fixation, vision breaks help with relieving the strain.*

➢ **Palming**

Cup your hands over your eyes with your elbows on your desk or knees. Concentrate on your breathing for 2 - 5 minutes, depending on how your eyes feel. ***Benefit:*** *This is an easy way to rest your eyes and take a relaxing break.*

3.8.2 Eye Exercises

Want to flex your visual muscles? Check out these simple eye exercises you can do to actually strengthen your eyesight.
(See: Quick Guides – Vitality Vision)

> ➤ Eight Tracing
> Imagine a figure 8 on its side 5 meters in front of you. Now trace along the figure 8 with your eyes slowly. Do this for 2 minutes in one direction and then 2 minutes in the reserve direction.
> ***Benefit:*** *This exercises your eye muscles and increases their flexibility.*

> ➤ Focus Switching
> Hold out your arm with your fist in a thumbs up position. Breath in as you focus on your thumb, then breath out and focus on an object 5 to 10 meters away. Repeat this for 2 to 5 minutes.
> ***Benefit:*** *This will strengthen the muscles in your eyes over time and improve your vision overall.*

> ➤ Zoom Focus
> Stretch out your arm with your fist in a thumbs up position. Focus on your thumb, now bring your thumb slowly closer to your face, all the time keeping focus on it. Stop once your thumb is 5inches in front of your face. Then move your thumb slowly back. Repeat this for 2 minutes. Benefit: This exercise will strengthen your focussing and your eye muscles in general.

3.9 Gamer Brain

Playing video games can be a fun and interesting pastime for people of all ages, however there are some ill side effects to playing video games such as Gamer Brain. This is a condition where the lines between reality and gaming begin to blur for those affected. What is important to understand is that there are simple and easy techniques for eliminating this potentially debilitating condition. By understanding that the brain is indeed the control center of the whole body, and that a healthy mind is one in the same with a healthy body anyone can recover. By reducing exposure to video games and other electronic gaming devices, an individual can quickly regain control of their mind and body.

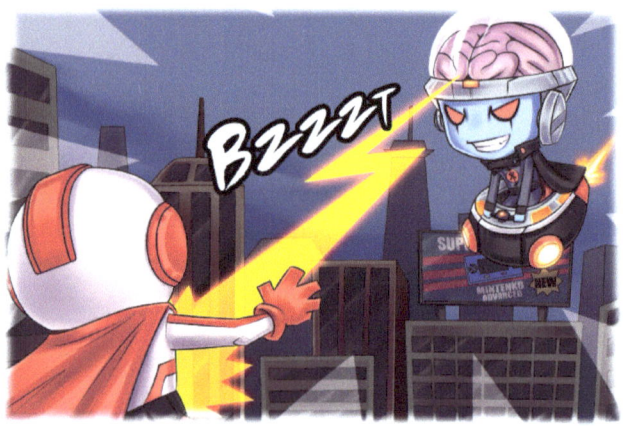

Renewing and Refreshing to the Mind, Body and Soul
Because video games can be sensational and intense they can quickly increase the heart rate and create conditioned responses in the human body. With this in mind one of the first things an individual can do after reducing their exposure to video games is to learn techniques in meditation and breathing. In its simplest form meditation is a way to become aware and conscious of one's breathing patterns. By intentionally focusing on the breathing and deliberately clearing the mind of all extraneous thoughts someone with a Gamer brain condition can work their way back to a healthy mind and body. The relaxation associated with meditation is renewing and refreshing to the mind, body and soul.

Meditation and Yoga

Meditation, when done correctly can rejuvenate and energize the human body beyond compare. Other active forms of meditation like yoga are also effective in rejuvenating the mind and body. In both meditation and yoga the intention is the same, to allow one to reconnect with their body and turn their focus away from distractions such as video games and other electronic screen-based activities. In addition, developing the habit of reading inspiring and uplifting books and other written material is a good way to give the mind a healthy dose of intellectual nutrition.

Positive and Healthy Thoughts

Advanced stages of Gamer Brain can severely distort one's perception of reality. That is why as a healthy alternative it is important to expose the brain to positive and healthy thoughts. Other factors that can have an impact on one's overall outlook on life include proper diet. When one is heavily engrossed in video games and other similar activities, proper diet and nutrition tend to take a backseat. When an individual turns the corner and begins to live a healthier and more fulfilled life they can begin to focus on a more healthy way of eating. Avoiding processed foods, sugary foods and caffeine to name a few is a good place to begin. When activities such as meditation, inspirational reading and proper nutrition are all combined together an individual can quickly return to a balanced way of life. This balanced lifestyle of healthy mind and healthy body along with a winning attitude is how to live a truly happy and successful life.

4. Become a Professional Gamer

You might have heard someone joke about what it would be like to play video games for a living, but there are people out there doing just that. Even though many people see video games has just another idle recreational activity, there exists an entire professional gaming scene where people do what they love and more importantly, get paid big bucks while doing it.

Becoming a professional gamer might seem like an easy gig to break into, but it's actually a lot harder than it seems on the surface. The learning curve can be steep, as you'll be squaring off with people who spent countless hours a day practicing and sharpening their gaming skills for tournaments and exhibitions. However, you should let that discourage you from pursuing what you love most, especially if you're extraordinarily passionate about it.

7. Steps to Becoming a Professional Gamer

These seven steps form a basic guideline for becoming a professional gamer. Once you have these seven steps down pat, you'll be able to turn a recreational activity you love into a fruitful career.

1. **Practice with the Right Game**

   Being a professional gamer means spending lots of time honing your gaming skills. That means you'll often spend eight or more hours a day playing the same game over and over for practice. You'll find yourself working on one or two particular aspects of your game play just to gain the advantage over your opponents.

   Practice makes perfect, but it's easy to get bored and lose discipline if you're playing a game you're just not into. That's why it's a good idea to find a game you really love to play that is also played on a professional level.

2. **Know your Environment**

Knowing the game like the back of your hand involves more than just knowing how to beat the game. Studying the game environment can mean the difference between success and failure.

"With non-Competition Games;
Don't always play to win, take time to test out ideas."

For example, an FPS game requires you to know where all of the possible camping spots and chokepoints are on the map. Knowing which weapons are the most effective for the game type and environment, as well as which objects you can shoot through can give you a tremendous advantage over other players. These are basic examples; with any game become inquisitive with all aspects of a game.

3. **Be Part of the Community**
    Each game has its own professional gamer community and being a part of that community gives you access to a wide range of information and support. By joining up with a gaming community, you can trade strategies, participate in critiques and enjoy in-depth discussions you might miss out on by being on the outside. Don't forget about outside input from friends, as it can also help your gaming skills tremendously as you break into the professional ranks.

4. **Gamer Health and Nutrition**
    Professional gaming is often seen as a sedentary lifestyle that unfortunately promotes poor diet and exercise habits. There is a bit of truth to this, as being planted in front of a gaming console and television for hours at a time just to take a toll on a person's health and well-being.

    Developing a nutritious diet and exercise regimen is essential for staying healthy and fit, especially for professional gamers. For instance, starting out with a healthy breakfast is one of the most important things you can do for your body. Professional gamers should avoid greasy foods, snacks and sodas laden with caffeine.

"Your mind and body are all part of the gaming experience;
you need both of these to be efficient and effective."

For a real challenge, Take on the **"Vitality Challenge"** and improve your overall gaming experience and ability.

5. **Build a Team**

   Once you get going on the road to professional Gamerdom, you'll want to have a team of fellow players and supporters that are willing to stand behind you every step of the way. You can start your own gaming guild and invite people with similar skills and aspirations. You'll essentially be creating your very own community to network and practice with.

   "To Lead a Team, you will need to be a Leader."

6. **Make a Name for Yourself**

   No one is going to know who you are unless you get out there and make a name for yourself. Participating in gaming tournaments and networking throughout the gaming community are two ways you can make yourself known in the professional gaming world.

Depending on where you live, you can find plenty of local gaming tournaments on a monthly basis. Some of these tournaments charge money for entry - this is to weed out some of the not-so-serious players right off the bat. You'll want to stick with tournaments offering free admission before moving up to ones requiring entry fees.

7. **Market Yourself**

Social media offers plenty of wonderful opportunities to market yourself to a wide audience both within and outside of the country. Keep in mind that you are your own brand and in order for your brand to stand out, you have to take proactive steps towards marketing that brand.

"Be your Game Avatar in Life."

Losing isn't the end - it's something that'll happen to you a lot as you start out. That's the most important thing that budding professional Gamers should always keep in mind. Learning how to keep your cool under pressure is an important aspect of professional gaming. After all, cooler heads do prevail in the long run. You can't win all of your games and any loss should be treated as something you can learn from and ultimately improve upon.

5. Quick Guides

HABIT CREATION

1. Plan what Habit to Create

- What habit/s do you want to create?
- Which of those habits would provide the most benefit to you right now?
- Start with only 1 or 2 habits to begin with.

"Trying to do everything, you will end up doing nothing."

2. Write Down the Habit / Goal

- *Write down the specific goal you want to achieve from doing the Habit.*
- *The act of writing stimulates sectors in the brain and imprints it on your mind better than just saying it would.*

3. Make it Visible

- Put your Habit and Goal somewhere you will see everyday

4. Make yourself Accountable

- Declare to the world what you will achieve (family, friends, etc.)

5. Commitment

- Commit to at least 30 days (90 days preferred), as studies have shown that it takes at least 21 times of doing something in a row to form a lasting habit.

6. Repeat (Go to Step 1)

www.VitalityForGamers.com

Vitality Challenge (Active)

Breakfast
Eat Fruit Only for Breakfast and up until Midday.

Gamer Snacks
Eat Fruit, Nuts and other healthy options for Gaming snacks.

Lunch/Dinner
Vegetables and Salad to make up 75% of your meals.

Fitness
Fat Burning Jog (or Brisk Walk) for 30 minutes, 5 days a week.

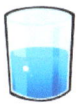

Drink Healthy
Drink Water and Fresh Juice.
(Reduce Soft-drinks, Coffee and Alcohol consumption)

Posture / Core Strength
Have good Gaming Posture and strengthen your core.
Do Yoga, Pilates or Core Strengthening exercises at least twice a week.

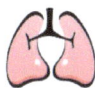

Oxygen
Do the 'Vitality Breath' daily to assist with your body's health.

Eye Sight
Take Eye Breaks and do Eye Exercises daily, especially when Gaming.

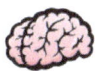

Brain
Relax, Meditate, have Positive and Healthy Thoughts

www.VitalityForGamers.com

VITALITY BREATH

1. Breath In for a ratio of 1

2. Hold your Breath for a ratio of 4

3. Breath out for a ratio of 2

4. Repeat the above steps 5 times

Example:

- As an example, if you breathe in for 5 seconds, you would hold your breath for 20 seconds and then breathe out for 10 seconds.

- Make sure you are relaxed during this and as you improve, increase the amount of time from 5 seconds.

- Make sure you always breathe at a pace you are comfortable with, if you are straining to hold your breath, then reduce the number of seconds.

www.VitalityForGamers.com

GAMER WEIGHT LOSS

1. Burn More Calories

- Burn more calories than you consume
- Add more physical activity to your day
- Avoid convenience, aim for inconvenience
- Don't Game, Eat and Sleep in the same room

2. Fat Burning Jog

- Jog or brisk walk for 30 minutes at least 3 days a week
- Casual Challenge (Unfit or new to jogging)
  Heart rate range: (170 minus your Age) to (180 minus your Age)
  Add 5 if you have jogged before and add 10 if you are fit.

3. Good Nutrition

- Eat more Vegetables, Salad, Fruit, seeds and beans
- Eat Fish at least one a week
- Reduce Red Meat intake
- Reduce starchy carbohydrates intake (Bread, Pasta etc.)

4. Drink Water

- Drink 8 Glasses of water a day (Pure Water)
- Eat more watery foods to assist with water intake
- Hunger can mimic thirst, so drink water first if feeling hungry

5. Sleep

- Ensure you receive 7 to 9 hours of sleep each day

www.VitalityForGamers.com

Top 12 Healthy Gamer Tips

1. Pre-Game Nutrition
Have a healthy meal prior to long gaming sessions.

2. Pre-Game Exercise
Exercise, jog or take a walk prior to gaming.

3. Take Breaks
Take breaks, stretch, walk around and focus on distant objects

4. Time Keeper
Have a clock visible so you do not lose track of time.

5. Drink Water
Drink water to keep your body hydrated.

6. Rage Reduction
Breath, learn to relax and organise your time for when you play games.

7. Spawn/Level Loading Exercises
Do push-ups, weights or dance while you wait (loading or spawning).

8. Glare reduction
Reduce glare from TV/Monitor (Keep away from direct light source).

9. Sit-Standing Desk
Use standing desk, or ensure you do not sit for long periods.

10. Good Posture
If sitting, make sure your back is supported and you have a body posture.

11. Healthy Snacks
Have healthy options such as Soaked Almond Nuts

12. Level up from being a NOOB
Learn the games environment/dynamics etc...

www.VitalityForGamers.com

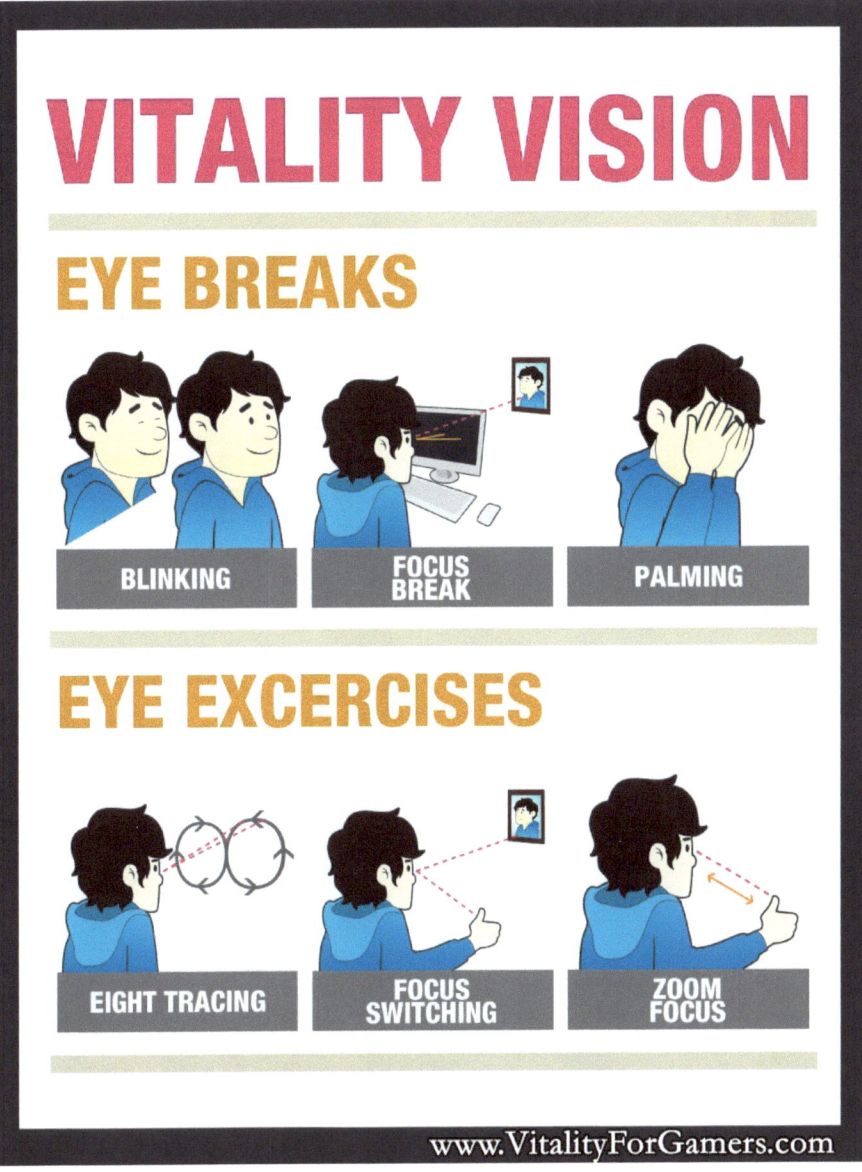

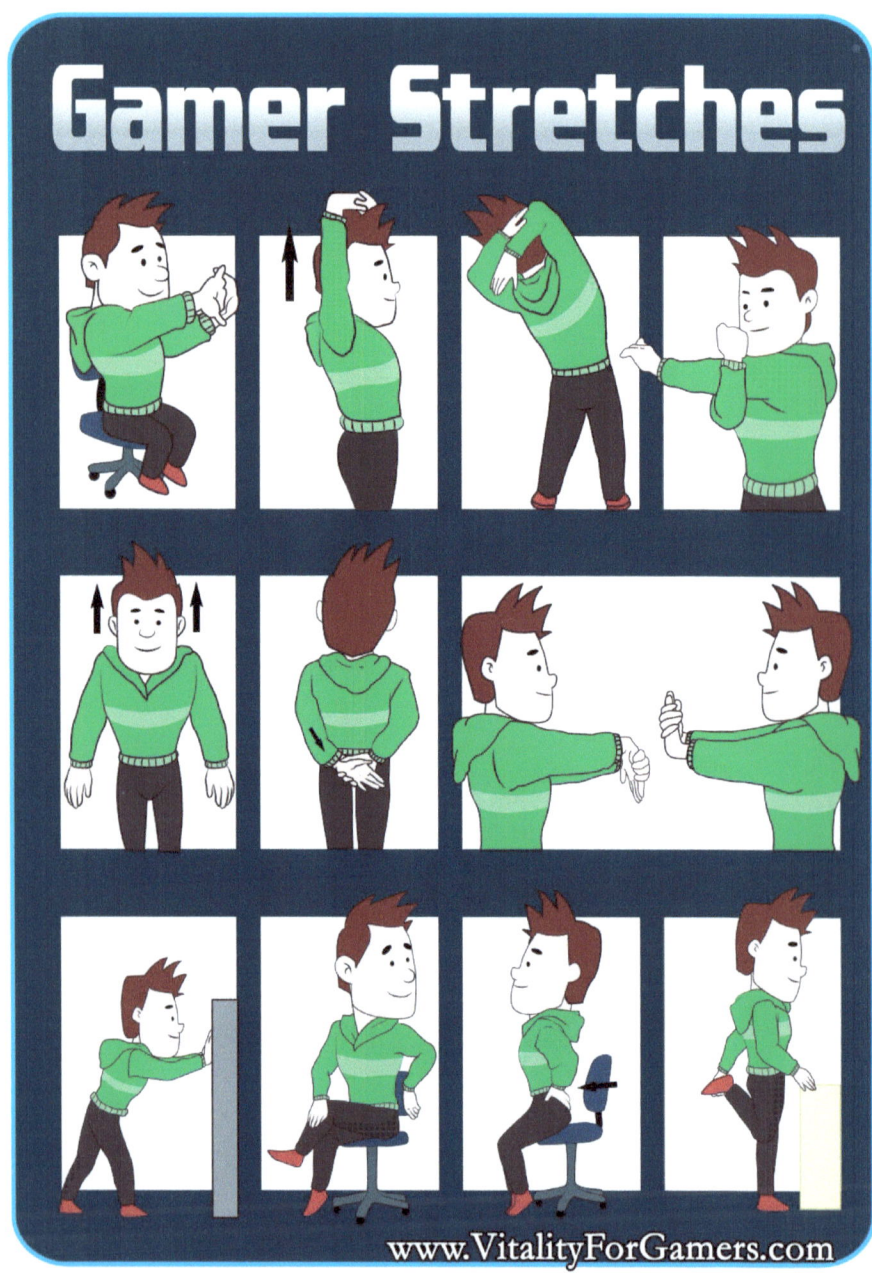

6. References

http://www.vitalityforgamers.com
National Institute of Neurological Disorders and Stroke:
http://www.ninds.nih.gov/disorders/carpal_tunnel/detail_carpal_tunnel.htm
University of Michigan: http://web.eecs.umich.edu/~cscott/rsi.html
NHS: http://www.nhs.uk/Conditions/Repetitive-strain-injury/Pages/Introduction.aspx
Repetitive Strain Injury.org: http://www.repetitivestraininjury.org.uk/
MFL Occupational Health Centre:
http://www.mflohc.mb.ca/fact_sheets_folder/repetitive_strain_injury.html
American Optometric Association: http://www.aoa.org/x5253.xml
WebMD: http://www.webmd.com/eye-health/computer-vision-syndrome
Mashable.com: http://mashable.com/2011/08/06/eyestrain-infographic/
Medscape: http://emedicine.medscape.com/article/1229858-overview
http://psych.wisc.edu/csgreen/brains_on_gamesNRN.pdf
http://healthland.time.com/2009/08/18/playing-too-many-video-games-is-bad-for-you-too-grown-ups/
http://www.sptimes.com/News/010301/Hillsborough/Father_guilty_in_deat.shtmlhttp://www.olganon.org/
http://thoughts.rockhymas.com/post/573231160/the-6-changes-habit-creation-technique-in-action
http://liveboldandbloom.com/04/self-improvement/habit-creation-for-beginners
http://www.pickthebrain.com/blog/8-reasons-why-you-fail-at-creating-new-habits/
http://johnstepper.com/2012/07/14/its-about-time-how-changing-a-keystone-habit-at-work-might-change-everything/
http://www.huffingtonpost.com/charles-duhigg/the-power-of-habit_b_1304550.html
http://www.kerenthrelfall.com/2012/04/04/simple-inspiration-keystone-habits/
http://johnstepper.com/2012/07/14/its-about-time-how-changing-a-keystone-habit-at-work-might-change-everything/
http://www.pickthebrain.com/blog/5-ways-to-change-a-habit/
http://www.vitalityforgamers.com/Vitality-Challenge/Gamer-Snacks-Fruit-and-Nuts.php
http://livingwithanerd.com/the-healthy-gamer-snacks-and-beverages-part-ii/
http://familyfitness.about.com/od/nutrition/a/halftime_snacks.htm
http://www.gadchick.com/blog/healthy-gaming-healthy-and-yummy-snacks-for-gaming/
http://www.hearthealthyonline.com/healthy-recipes/appetizer-recipes/game-day-snacks_1.html
http://startcooking.com/top-23-snacks-for-all-night-gaming
http://www.self-improvement-mentor.com/what-is-a-habit.html
http://liveboldandbloom.com/04/self-improvement/habit-creation-for-beginners
http://www.entrepreneur.com/blog/224079
http://www.lifehack.org/articles/productivity/18-tricks-to-make-new-habits-stick.html
http://johnstepper.com/2012/07/14/its-about-time-how-changing-a-keystone-habit-at-work-might-change-everything/
http://www.amazon.com/The-Power-Habit-What-Business/dp/1400069289/
http://www.kerenthrelfall.com/2012/04/04/simple-inspiration-keystone-habits/
http://stress.about.com/od/lowstresslifestyle/ss/healthy_habits.htm
http://www.forbes.com/sites/insertcoin/2012/03/30/the-10-steps-to-becoming-a-pro-gamer/
http://www.ehow.com/how_2129923_become-professional-gamer.html
http://www.alteredgamer.com/gaming/63880-how-to-become-a-professional-gamer/
http://www.joystiq.com/2005/11/17/tips-on-becoming-a-pro-gamer/

http://www.heraldsun.com.au/technology/from-n00b-to-pro-meet-the-people-who-quit-their-day-jobs-to-become-gamers/story-fn5izo02-1226462242269

http://www.mayoclinic.com/health/medical/IM00594

http://news.discovery.com/human/glass-water-weight-loss.html

http://www.boston.com/bostonglobe/editorial_opinion/oped/articles/2011/05/14/gamer_brain/

http://www.bbc.co.uk/news/health-15720178

http://www.osha.gov/SLTC/etools/computerworkstations/positions.html

http://www.betterhealth.vic.gov.au/bhcv2/bhcarticles.nsf/pages/Posture

7. Vitality For Gamers

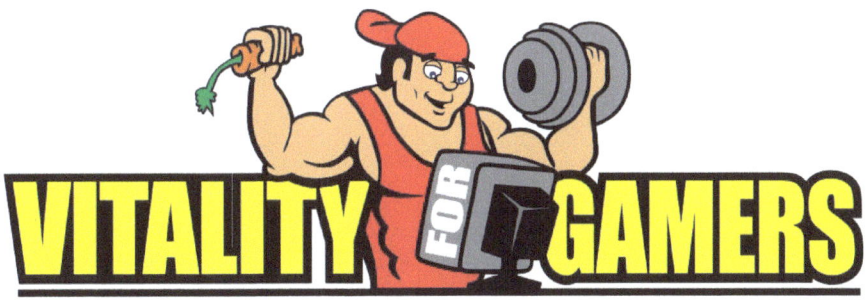

Our goal is to give computer game players increased reflexes, endurance and longevity for better gaming. In essence creating a healthier gamer lifestyle and changing the gamer stereotype.

"Find out what is possible when you become your Gaming Avatar in real life by doing the Vitality Challenge..."

Join the Vitality For Gamers community and make a difference in the world. Create vitality in your life, improve your health, well-being and increase the demands for healthy food and activities in your local community.

Join Us for the Greater Good!

www.VitalityForGamers.com

Short Website URL Version:

www.VFORG.com